The Atkins Diet Weight Loss Guide

Low Carb Recipes and Diet Plan for Beginner

by FlatBelly Queens

Published in Great Britain by:

FlatBelly Queens
345 Old Street
London
EC1V 9LE

© Copyright 2016 – Flatbelly Queens

ISBN-13: {978-1533319869}
ISBN-10: {1533319863}

Table of Contents

Introduction:

You've tried losing weight, but have failed. You hate to count calories or to feel that you have to restrict how much you eat, so you are always hungry. You are beginning to think that there is no hope for you.

Don't give up quite yet, because there is hope, on the Atkins diet. Many people have found the answer to their weight loss question when they start to follow the low-carb plan advocated in the Atkins diet. Instead of counting calories, you count the net carbs that you eat. You don't have to feel deprived, and you are encouraged to eat enough food so that you feel satiated and full.

This book will describe the Atkins diet in detail, including the four phases of the diet, the foods that you can eat on each phase, and even some recipes that you can try. All your questions will be answered in this book. By the time you are finished, you will have all the information and the tools that you need to succeed on the Atkins diet. You can lose weight fast. In fact, many people report being able to lose up to 30 pounds in 30 days!

So what are you waiting for? This book has the answers that you are looking for.

Chapter 1:

What is the Atkins Diet?

The Atkins Diet was developed by Dr. Robert Atkins, a cardiologist, in 1972. At that time, he released the book *Dr. Atkin's Diet Revolution*. However, the diet did not really catch on in the 1970s. It wasn't until 2002, when he released a revised version of the book, *Dr. Atkins New Diet Revolution*, that people began to pay attention. So many people who didn't have success with typical diets which require restricting calories found that they were able to lose the weight they so desperately wanted to by doing Akins.

But what is the Atkins Diet? Basically, Atkins found that when you cut out most carbohydrates and sugars, but didn't restrict other foods, people lost weight. It's not about completely cutting out carbs, but includes eating only those carbs that are nutrient dense. His diet is based on the premise that people who cut carbs and sugars, but are able to eat anything else, will lose weight. And the results have shown this to be true. People who start on the Atkins Diet have lost up to 30 pounds in the first thirty days! The results bear themselves out. Be willing to cut out carbs and sugars, while not restricting anything else that you eat, and you can lose weight. The research has proven this.

How does this work? Basically, the idea behind the Atkins diet is that the body has two different options that they can use for fuel: either sugar from the foods you eat, or stored fats in the body. The body will use simple sugars and carbs first, because it is the easiest to utilize. If you stop eating sugars and carbohydrates, which are turned into sugars in the body, that only leaves one fuel source for your body, the fats that you have already stored. Because sugars aren't available, the body will start to metabolize the stored fats, especially those fats around the belly area, to fuel the body. And you lose weight. It is really that simple.

Of course, the diet is a little more complex than this. The diet is broken down into four phases. The phases are based on the amount of net carbs that you eat.

Net carbs are very simple to calculate. To find the net carbs in any food, take the total number of carbohydrates listed on the nutrition info minus the amount of dietary fiber (both these units are generally shown in grams on a nutrition label), and this will equal the net carbs. Dietary fiber does not get processed as sugars in the body and have a negligible effect on the blood sugar levels in the system, so they are not necessary to cut.

Now that you understand net carbs, here is the four phases of the Atkins diet system.

Phase one allows only 20-25 grams

of net carbs per day and does not allow any type of carbohydrate-based foods, getting the net carbs you eat mostly from the vegetables in your diet. This is also often called the Induction phase, meaning that your body is being inducted into eating low carbs. This is the most restrictive phase of the diet, and can sometimes be tough on people who are not used o eating so few carbs. Of course, any change in diet can be difficult at first, but once you see the changes to your body and how quickly you will lose weight, you won't feel so deprived. Most people will stay in the induction phase for at least two weeks, but if you have a lot of weight to lose, you can stay in it for much longer.

Phase 2 can be started at least two weeks after phase 1, although most people wait until they are within 15 pounds of their goals weight. That means if you have a lot to lose, you won't move to phase 2 for a long time. Some people do choose to move to phase 2 earlier, but the weight will come off more slowly. You will still see weight loss, however. Phase 2 allows 25-50 grams of net carbs per day, and adds foods such as whole grains and high carb fruits.

In Phase 3, you are allowed to eat from 50-80 grams of net carbs. You can start this phase when you are within 5 pounds of your goal weight.

Phase 4 is also called the lifetime maintenance phase, which is where you can go from 80-100 grams of net carbs. This is the phase that you should eat at for the rest of your life to maintain your weight loss.

After all, you want to find a happy medium between being able to eat foods that you enjoy and keeping weight off. Atkins will help you progress between very restricted net carbs to finding a balance for your body to have healthy carbs added while still maintaining your weight loss.

The four phases will be discussed more fully in Chapter 5.

Now that you have a basic understanding of what the Atkins diet is, let's move on and discuss the benefits of the Atkins diet.

Chapter 2: Benefits of Following Atkins

There are many benefits to following the Atkins diet. This chapter will discuss those benefits.

First and foremost, you will lose weight quickly on Atkins. Because much of the obesity epidemic in this country is due to eating refined carbohydrates and sugar, by eliminating these things from your diet, you will start to lose weight almost immediately. You can lose up to 30 pounds in 30 days on the Atkins diet! This, of course, is why most people go on the Atkins diet. They haven't been able to lose weight on any other system, but can with Atkins.

But beyond weight loss, there are some great benefits to following this diet. First, several studies have shown that following Atkins can reduce the risk for the contributing factors for heart disease, including lowering blood pressure, lowering cholesterol and triglyceride levels, and decreasing inflammation in the body, which has been shown to increase the chance of developing heart disease.

Second, losing weight can reduce the risk for some kinds of cancer. Studies have shown that people who have lost weight decrease their risk of colon and breast cancer, even in survivors who are at a risk of recurrence.

Low-carb diets such as Atkins have been shown to reduce the risk of cognitive impairments, such as diseases like Alzheimer's. If you eat low-carb, you may be reducing your risk for dementias.

If you have diabetes, going low-carb can be good for you. Many different studies have verified that following a low-carb diet, such as Atkins can decrease the symptoms of diabetes, improve the problem of insulin resistance, and can help with different metabolic disorders.

Studies have shown that the risk for women developing Polycystic Ovary Syndrome (PCOS), which is an endocrine disorder that can affect women in their child-bearing years that causes small cysts to form on their ovaries. It has been shown that this disorder is associated with obesity and insulin resistance, both of which can effectively be reduced by following a low-carb diet.

Low-carb diets were also shown to improve the problem of daytime sleepiness in people who suffer from narcolepsy, a disorder where people uncontrollably fall asleep during the day.

As you can see, there are many benefits to following the Atkins diet. If you suffer from any of these diseases, besides losing weight, you could see some significant improvements in a variety of medical disorders!

The next chapter will discuss some of the biggest questions that people who are interested in following the Atkins diet may have.

Chapter 3: Atkins Diet FAQ

In this chapter, we will answer the top questions that people have about following the Atkins diet. Once you are done with this chapter, you should know everything you need in order to feel comfortable starting the Atkins diet. It is natural to be a little apprehensive when making a big change, and we want you to feel comfortable with this.

Isn't it dangerous to lose weight so quickly?

Because of the way the Atkins diet works on the body, you will lose weight very quickly. At first, it could be both fat and water weight that you are losing. When your body takes in fewer carbohydrates, you will stop retaining water, so much of the weight you lose in the first week will be this water that your body no longer needs. After a few days on the diet, however, you will start losing fat.

The only time it is dangerous to lose weight so quickly is if you are doing one of two things. The first is if you are starving yourself to try to lose. This is sometimes a problem with calorie restricted diets because you may not be taking enough food in, which will cause you to lose lean muscle mass, not fat. But, if you follow Atkins appropriately, take in adequate calories, and eat regular meals, this is not a problem. Second, if you are feeling sick, weak, fatigued, or dizzy, you could have a problem. It could be because you are not taking in enough water after how much you will lose on the diet, or because you aren't eating enough. As long as you do not have either of these two problems, it is not a problem to lose weight quickly on this diet.

Can you cat carbs on Atkins?

There is a misunderstanding about the Atkins diet that is prevalent which says that you cannot eat any carbohydrates on the Atkins diet. This is not true, however. Even in phase 1, 20-25 grams of net carbs are allowed. Most people, however, do not realize that Atkins moves through phases where more carbs are gradually added. They mistakenly believe that phase 1 is the entire diet, which is not true. Also, there are some carbs allowed in phase 1. It has never been a no carb diet.

Don't you eat too much fat on the Atkins diet?

Because you are cutting out most carbs from your diet (especially in phase 1), you will naturally eat more fats. However, Atkins diet promotes the eating of healthy fats, which have benefits for you. These fats include saturated fats that are found in lean animal protein, polyunsaturated fats in different types of vegetable oils, and monounsaturated fats that are found in foods like olive oil and avocados. Many fats are given the bad wrap in the press, but in reality, the body needs fats to survive and several different fats have been shown to have health benefits.

How long can I stay in Phase 1 of the Atkins diet?

Everyone should stay in phase 1 at least two weeks. This will help your body move into a state of ketosis, which is where you are burning fat from your body stores to utilize for energy. This is the goal of the diet. Because this is the primary phase of weight loss, most people stay in this phase much longer than two weeks.

As long as you have these thing occurring, you can stay in Phase 1 as long as you need. Most people stay in Phase 1 until they are about 15 pounds from their goal weight. As long as your blood chemistry panels are normal, you feel good and your sleep and energy patterns are normal, and you are not bored on the diet, you can stay in phase one. Remember, phase 1 is the most restrictive of the phases in terms of what you can eat, so many people will choose to move into phase 2 more quickly so that they can eat a wider variety of food. You can still lose weight in phase 2, but it will be a little slower.

How do I know when to move into the next phase of the Atkins diet?

Generally, people move from phase 1 to phase 2 either when they are about 15 pounds of their weight loss goal, they are bored with the lack of variety of food in phase 1, or their body is telling them that they need to add more carbs to their diet. Phase 2 still allows for weight loss, but it is not as fast as phase 1.

Each week, you add about 5 grams of carbs to get from phase 2 to phase 3. To go from phase 3 to phase 4, you add 10 grams of carbs incrementally until you get to the point where you can maintain your weight loss.

Move to phase 3 when you are within 5 pounds of your goal weight. This phase will add a few more carbs to your diet and allow for even greater variety of food. Lastly, phase 4 is the lifetime maintenance phase. When you hit your goal weight, phase 4 will help you keep it off. This becomes your permanent way of eating and living. This will be discussed more thoroughly in the chapter on the four phases of Atkins.

Can vegetarians follow Atkins?

It is possible for vegetarians and vegans to lose weight on the Atkins diet. Most vegetarians choose to start the diet in phase 2 of the diet to allow for seeds and nuts, which provide both carbs and protein. Vegetarians can get plenty of protein from eggs, cheese, and soy products. Vegans can get protein from seeds, nuts, soy products, soy and rice cheeses, legumes, and high protein grains such as quinoa.

What can I do if I hit a plateau and just don't lose any more weight?

Some people will lose weight quickly, but then hit a plateau on the Atkins diet. Often this is because they moved too quickly through the phases and are eating too many carbs to effectively lose weight. If you find that your weight loss has stalled, here are a few things you can try:

- Decrease the number of net carbs in your diet from 5 to 120 grams. However, do not do this if you are still in phase 1.
- Increase the amount of fat you eat and decrease the amount of protein. This is true if you are eating more than 4 to 6 ounces of protein per serving.
- Make sure that there are no hidden carbs in your diet. These can be found frequently in processed foods, where sugars add to the carbohydrate total. Also, check things like salad dressings, which are often flavoured with sugar.

- Increase your activity level. Remember, any form of exercise will help you lose weight faster.
- Make sure that you are drinking enough water. If your body is dehydrated, it will retain water. Increase your water intake.
- Cut back on artificial sweeteners and cheese. Artificial sweeteners especially can cause the body to gain weight, even though they themselves do not contain any calories.
-

By doing a combination of these things, you will restart the weight loss process.

Can I drink alcohol on the Atkins diet?

During phase 1, you should not drink any alcohol. Many drinks, especially beers and wine, contain a great many carbs, so they are not allowed on phase 1. The problem with drinking is that your body will use the alcohol for fuel, rather than burning its own fat stores, so it does slow down your progress. Once you are in phase 2 and beyond, a glass of wine occasionally should not be a problem. Spirits such as scotch, rye, gin, and vodka are ok, as they do not contain carbs, but you cannot mix them with juices, tonic water, or sugary sodas, as all of these things contain sugars that will add to your carb count. You can mix with seltzer, diet tonics or diet sodas. If you find that drinking alcohol slows or stops your weight loss, you need to cut out alcohol from your diet completely.

How can artificial sweeteners inhibit weight loss?

Many studies have been done that show that artificial sweeteners have the same effect on insulin in the body as does regular sugar, causing spikes in blood sugar, which can slow or stop the progress of weight loss. By consuming artificial sweeteners, you may be inhibiting your body from entering into ketosis and losing weight. Atkins does not necessarily ban artificial sweeteners, but if you find that you are doing everything else right, yet still consuming these products, try cutting them out and seeing if that helps you restart your weight loss. The recommended artificial sweeteners on Atkins are sucralose, saccharine, or stevia. One packet of each contains one net carb.

Now that you have your basic questions about the Atkins diet answered, the next chapter will talk about the keys to finding success on the Atkins diet. After that, the following chapter will go into a more in-depth discussion about the four phases, what should be done in each, and the appropriate foods to eat.

Chapter 4: Keys to Success on Atkins

Some people find it fairly easy to cut back on carbs and have great success without any problems on the Atkins diet. Other people, however, have more difficulty switching to the Atkins diet. It can be a surprise to go from eating much of your caloric intake in carbs to moving to a very low-carb diet, but, with the following keys to success, you will be able to transition more smoothly.

First, make sure to make the best use of your net carbs. Remember, net carbs are the total number of carbohydrates in your food minus the dietary fiber. The remainder is the net carb for that food. Since fiber has almost no impact on your blood sugar, it is not necessary to cut down fiber. It is best to get your complete allotment of net carbs, especially in phase 1. Make sure you eat all your net carbs!

Second, make sure to eat plenty of vegetables. In phase 1, most of your net carbs (12 to 15 grams) will be found in the vegetables that you eat. The next chapter will talk more about what vegetables you should consume in each phase of the diet.

Make sure to keep salt in your diet. As your body transitions from carb burning for energy to fat burning, if you do not get enough salt, you may suffer from headaches, lightheadedness, cramps, or a feeling of weakness or lethargy. By making sure that there is adequate sodium intake, you should be able to avert these symptoms as your body adapts to the new way of eating.

Also, as important as salt, is to drink plenty of water. Most people go through life dehydrated and don't even know it. It is important to note that when you are dehydrated, it may feel like being hungry. This is one reason some people eat too much. Instead of eating when you get a sign of hunger pains, start with a glass of water. Also, there is an easy key to see if you are dehydrated: check the color of your urine. You want to make sure that your urine is a light yellow or clear. If your urine is dark, it means that you aren't getting enough liquid. You should get at least 64 ounces a day, but larger people and people who are very active will need more.

The next tip is to make sure that you eat plenty of protein. Protein has a way of filling you up longer. It takes longer to digest than simple carbs, so, when you get enough protein, you will feel fuller longer, which helps you stick to the plan (especially in the induction phase). Make sure to eat 4 to 6 ounces of protein with every meal.

Make sure to get enough fat to feel full. It can be difficult to have most of your diet be primarily fats and proteins because eating fat has gotten a bad rap in our society. However, eating fat will help you control your carb intake, and the fats that are recommended in the Atkins diet are actually good for you! Eating processed foods with a lot of fat is not necessarily a good thing, but eating fats from vegetable oils, olive oils, and lean meats are important. Just don't go overboard. You should make sure that you feel full after eating, but don't go overboard on eating fats.

Next, check all your foods for hidden carbs, especially if you are eating processed foods. Many things have sugars added for flavor, especially condiments such as ketchup, salad dressings, and others. Make sure you are aware of all these hidden carbs in your foods, use low-carb foods (and still read the label), and stay within your net carb count. You may be surprised by what you find when you become an expert label reader.

Watch your calorie counts. Although you don't have to count calories on the Atkins diet, it is important that you do not overeat either. If you follow Atkins but eat 3,000 calories a day, your body will have fats to burn for fuel from your food instead of your stored fat. And this will hinder your weight loss. Most women should eat between 1500 and 1800 calories and most men between 1800 and 2200 calories. Basically, your portions should be sensible, not humongous. You know when you get into a restaurant and they fill huge plates? Those portions are too big. Eating sensible portions will help you maintain a reasonable amount of food.

Make sure to stay moving. Regular exercise, even taking a walk, will help you lose weight faster. If you do no exercise, it will be harder for the weight to come off, no matter what diet plan you follow.

Another tip that many people have found especially helpful is to plan your foods beforehand. When you know what you are going to eat and when, it is easier to succeed on a diet. After all, you won't be surprised by that 3pm hunger strike that always made you want to go to the vending machine before. Now, when you have a sensible snack already ready for you to eat, you won't be tempted by junk. If you have planned for your food, you will be ready to face the day without fear of getting hungry.

One of the most important tips to follow on the Atkins diet is to track the foods you eat. This is especially important for tracking your net carbs. Study after study have found that people who track what they eat have greater success with a weight loss plan (any weight loss plan) than those who do not. So, keeping track of your food will do several things for you. First, it will help you to track your net carbs and make sure that you aren't eating more carbohydrates than you think you are. It will help you see patterns that you may not have noticed. If you aren't losing any weight, can you attribute it to a certain food? If you don't feel well, is it because you aren't getting enough protein? These things can be the difference between success and failure on any diet. Lastly, it will tell you if you are eating too much. After all, no matter what plan you are on, if you eat too much food, you will not be able to lose weight. It is as simple as that. So tracking can be the make-or-break habit for the diet.

If you follow these tips, the Atkins diet will be much easier to follow and you will have greater success as a result. And now that you have all the basic information, let's dive into exactly what each phase of the diet requires. This is the meat and potatoes of what Atkins is. Once you have read the next chapter, you will be ready to begin to create your healthier, happier life and lose the weight you have   been   struggling   with.

Chapter 5: The 4 Phases of Atkins

This chapter will go in depth in discussing each phase of the Atkins diet. Once you have ready this chapter, you should have all the information you need to begin and succeed on Atkins.

Phase 1: Induction

In phase 1, which is also known as the induction

phase of Atkins, you will shift your body from burning carbs for fuel to burning the stored fat in your body for fuel. This, of course, is the key to weight loss on the Atkins diet. When your body no longer gets adequate carbohydrates to burn for fuel from the food you eat, it will shift into a state called ketosis, where it starts to burn the fat that is already stored in the body. This is why it is important to cut carbs so drastically: your body will use carbohydrates for fuel first because it is the easiest for it to utilize. But, once carbs are not available, it will shift into ketosis and burn the fats your body already has stored. This is the key to weight loss.

To get your body into the ketosis stage, you should cut your net carbs down to 20 grams per day. This is the level at which almost everyone will go into ketosis and start burning body fat.

Most people will stay in phase 1 for at least two weeks, but often will stay in this phase for much longer. This is the part of the diet where the majority of weight loss will occur. Most people will stay in phase 1 until they are within approximately 15 pounds of their goal weight. This means that, if you have a great deal of weight to lose, you will stay in phase 1 for quite a while.

There are several things that you can do to make eating in phase 1 easier for you. It is recommended that you eat five or six small meals during the day so that you are not hungry. Most people can have success with three meals and two snacks in between. The theory behind this is that if you are not ever hungry, you will not be tempted to cheat on the diet. Of course, this means you will be eating less at every meal, but it gives you less time to experience hunger pangs. Also, when eating, make sure to get enough protein and fat. Each meal should have 4 to 6 ounces of protein, and adequate natural fats to feel satiated. Last, make sure that you consume all your carbs. By restricting carbs more than Atkins already does, you will feel hungry and will not lose weight any faster. So, it is imperative that you eat your 20 grams of net carbs every single day. Twelve to 15 grams will be in acceptable vegetables.

Foods that are acceptable and recommended for Phase 1 include:

- Fish: all kinds of fish, including salmon, sardines, herring, flounder, trout, cod, tuna, and halibut.
- Shellfish: Clams, crab, shrimp, squid, and lobster. You can eat mussels and oysters, but they have a higher carb content, so should be limited to 4 ounces of each per day.
- Poultry: All kinds of poultry can be eaten, including chicken, turkey, Cornish hens, duck, goose, pheasant, quail, and even ostrich!
- Meats: A variety of meats are included on the Atkins diet, including beef, lamb, pork, veal, and venison. Bacon and ham are also allowed, but be sure that they are not cured with added sugars,

which will add to your carb count. The meats that you should avoid are cold cuts and other meats that contain nitrates, as foods that are cured with nitrates may have hidden carbs that you are not aware of.

- Eggs: Eggs are a great staple to the Atkins diet and can be prepared in almost any way that you like. You can also add vegetables, cheese, and herbs to eggs.

- Fats and oils: There are many fats and oils that you can keep in your diet, and will help you to feel full for longer. Such things include butter, mayonnaise (check for hidden sugars), olive oil, and any type of vegetable oil, such as canola oil, sunflower oil, soybean, walnut, grape seed, and sesame oils.

- Liquids: There are plenty of liquids that you can take on the Atkins diet. Of course, you should start with water, drinking at least 64 ounces a day. This can include filtered water, mineral water, spring water, and tap water. Other liquids you can have is clear broth (as long as it has no added sugars), club soda, cream (no more than 3 tablespoons per day), coffee, tea (do not add sugar to these), diet soda (check the carb count), zero-calorie flavoured seltzer, unflavoured soy or almond milk, and lemon or lime juice (up to 3 tablespoons per day. Make sure to note and count any net carbs that are in these drinks.

- Cheese: Cheese contains about a gram of carbs per ounce, so you must count it, but you can have 3 to 4 ounces of cheese per day. This includes feta cheese, Swiss, parmesan, cream cheese, mozzarella, Gouda, cheddar, goat cheese, and bleu cheese.

- Vegetables: Several times in this books, we have talked about making sure to get enough vegetables in this diet. The vegetables that you can have in phase 1 are known as foundation vegetables. These are listed with the amount of net carbs per half cup raw in parentheses after unless otherwise noted: alfalfa sprouts (0), chicory greens (0.1), endive (0.1), escarole (0.1), watercress (0.1), arugula (0.2), radishes (1 radish, 0.2) spinach (0.2), bok choy (0.4), lettuce (0.5), turnip greens (cooked, 0.6), radicchio (0.7), mushrooms (0.8), celery (one stalk, 1.0), collard greens (cooked, 1.0), spinach (1.0), sauerkraut (1.2), avocado (half fruit, 1.3), onion (2 tablespoon, 1.5), zucchini (cooked, 1.5), cucumber (1.5), cauliflower (cooked 1.7), broccoli (cooked 1.8), rhubarb (1.8) Swiss chard (cooked 1.8), asparagus (6 stalks 1.9), green bell pepper (2.2), eggplant (cooked 2.3), kale (cooked 2.4), tomato (1 small 2.5), yellow squash (cooked 2.6), cabbage (cooked 2.7), green beans (cooked 2.9), red bell pepper (3.0), leeks or shallots (cooked 2 tablespoons 3.4), spaghetti squash (cooked 4.0), garlic (2 tablespoons 5.3), snow peas (cooked 5.4), and tomato (cooked 8.6). Remember that you should eat 12 to 15 grams of your net carbs in vegetables. This will help you feel full for longer, as the fiber will keep you satiated. It is important to measure out your vegetables so that you aren't getting more net carbs than you think you are.

- Salad dressings: You can eat salad dressing, but make sure that you are aware of the net carbs that are in them. Red wine vinegar is your best bet, as it has no net carbs in a tablespoon. Caesar dressing only has 1 gram net carbs in 2 tablespoons. Check the label of your dressing to figure out your net cards.

- As a side note, if you are staying in the induction phase for longer than two weeks, you can switch out 3 grams of net carb of vegetables for 3 grams of net carbs in nuts or seeds. Just make sure not to allow your net carbs from foundation vegetables fall below 12 grams.

-

Now that you know what you can eat in phase 1 of the Atkins diet, you are ready to get going.

As stated before, you can choose to stay in phase 1 to lose the bulk of your weight, or you may choose to move to phase 2, which will still allow you to lose weight, but at a slightly slower pace. Once you are ready to transition to phase 2, start with switching out vegetables for nuts, as described above. The next step to transition is to add 5 grams of net carbs to your diet. Move on to phase 2 to find out more about this.

Phase 2: Balancing

In phase 2, also called the balancing phase, you begin to start adding carbs to your diet. You will slowly add foods that you had cut out in phase 1 and begin adding them back slowly, one by one. This way, you will be able to tell if a specific food is causing weight gain or triggering cravings for foods that may cause you to gain weight.

Most people will stay on phase two until they are about 10 pounds from their goal weight. Some people do choose to do most of their weight loss in phase 2, while others will do so in phase 1. This is based on what you are most comfortable with.

When you transition to phase 2, you add five grams of net carbs to your diet. So you start phase 2 at 25 grams of net carbs per day. You continue to add carbs until your weight loss levels off, and then you back off a bit. You will add 5 grams of net carbs per week (or more, some do it biweekly or monthly) until you reach the point that weight loss stops, then dial it back 5 grams. This number could be anywhere from 30 grams to 80 grams of net carbs, and has to do with age, gender, activity level, and other personal factors. Continue to get at least 12-15 grams of net carbs in foundation vegetables listed in phase 1.

When reintroducing foods, make sure to do so one by one to see how they react with your system. That way, if a specific food causes a craving, you know what food is doing it and that you should cut it out.

Foods that you can add in phase 2 include:

- Dairy: At this point, other dairy foods can be added including: mozzarella cheese, yogurt (Greek or regular, plain and unsweetened), whole milk, ricotta cheese, 2% cottage cheese, and heavy cream. Make sure to check the nutrition label for serving size and net carbs.
- Nuts: This is when nuts and seeds are added back into the diet. These include 6 Brazil nuts (1.4 g net carbs), macadamia (10 nuts, 1.4), sunflower seeds (2 tablespoons, 1.5), walnuts (12 nuts, 1.7), almonds (24 nuts 2.2), pistachios (2 tablespoons 3.0) peanuts (2 tablespoons 3.8), pecans (2 tablespoons 3.8), and cashews (2 tablespoons 5.1).
- Fruits: now is a good time to start adding berries and melons back into your diet. Each fruit is listed with its net carbs for a ¼ cup serving: blackberries(1.6), raspberries (1.7), cranberries (1.9), strawberries (2.4), cantaloupe (2.9), honeydew (3.5), gooseberries (3.9), boysenberries and blueberries (4.5).
- Legumes: at this point you can also add a variety of canned beans, including lentils, kidney beans,

lima beans, pinto beans, black beans, navy beans, and chickpeas.

As always, make sure to check the nutrition information on the package for the net carbs.

Of course, you can continue to eat any foods from the phase 1 list as you move through to phase 2. Each phase builds on the last, so it gives you more variety to your diet.

You should stay in phase 2 until you have reached about 10 pounds from your goal weight. Once you are at this point, you are ready to start transitioning to phase 3, which will begin to teach you how to eat for a lifetime.

Phase 3: Pre-Maintenance

Once you are within 10 pounds of your goal weight, you can transition into phase 3. You will stay in phase 3 until you have reached your desired weight and maintained it for a month. The purpose of phase 3 is to shed those last few pounds and to start to figure out how many carbs you can safely add back to your diet without gaining weight. Like in phase 2, you will slowly increase your carb intake, but in phase 3 you will go up by 10 grams of net carbs per week (or biweekly, or monthly). You can continue to up your carb intake as long as you are able to lose weight, or maintain your desired weight goal. Some people do continue to add carbs in 5-gram increments if 10 seems to be too much.

Don't be afraid to drop your net carb intake by ten grams if you stop losing or start gaining. The point of this phase is to find out how many net carbs you can eat without gaining weight. This is your carb tolerance. After all, now that you have lost almost all of the weight you desired, you need to find a way to maintain that weight loss.

Besides watching for weight gain or a stall in loss, you need to be aware, as you add back more foods, what foods cause you to have uncontrollable hunger or cravings. Those foods are probably something that you will need to eliminate from your diet. You can cut it out for a week then try to add it back again. If you cannot tolerate it, you know that is a food that you should stay away from.

Foods that you can start adding back, one at a time, in phase 3 include:

- Starchy vegetables: Each of these is measured in ½ cup servings unless otherwise listed: carrots (1 medium 4.1), rutabaga (5.9), beets (6.8), peas (7.0), acorn squash (7.6), sweet potato (9.9), parsnips (10.2), potato (half of small 13.1), and corn (14.9).
- Fruit: At this stage, you can add more fruits to your diet. These include coconut (1/2 cup 2.5), fresh figs (1 fruit 4.5), cherries (1/4 cup 5.3), watermelon (1/2 cup 5.5), papaya (1/2 cup 6.6), plum (1 medium 6.6), raisins (1 tablespoon 6.8), guava (1/2 cup 7.4), apple (1/2 fruit 7.9), clementine (1 fruit 7.6), kiwi (1 fruit 8.1), grapefruit (1/2 fruit 8.9), pineapple (1/2 cup 9.7), small peach (10.5), red grapes (1/2 cup 13.0), navel orange (1 fruit 14.5), dates (3 fruit 15.8), small banana (1 fruit 20.4), and medium pear (1 fruit 21.0).
- Grains: in this phase of Atkins, you can start to add grains back into your diet. Just make sure to take note of the net carbs. The net carbs are not listed here, check the label of each individual grain that you eat. Those you can add include wheat

bran, wheat germ, oat bran, quinoa, whole wheat bread, steel cut or dry oatmeal, polenta, grits, whole wheat pasta, barley, millet, and rice.

How do you know that you are willing to transition to phase 4? If you can answer yes to these three questions, you can move on to the next phase, which is also called the maintenance phase:

Are you at your goal weight?

Has your weight remained constant for at least 4 weeks?

Are cravings and undue hunger not a problem anymore?

If you find that all three are true, you can move on to phase 4, the maintenance phase, where you settle into a lifetime eating pattern.

Phase 4: Maintenance

Once you are in phase 4, or the maintenance phase, you are doing what you should for the rest of your life. You will maintain your weight loss by developing your permanent way of living in this phase. If you start to gain weight, you can always cut back your total net carbs.

By the time you are in phase 4, you have been gradually increasing your carb intake to find your optimal balance, you know what foods you should avoid because they cause cravings or hunger, you have learned to be aware of your hunger cues and how to deal with them before entering into a food crisis, you know which foods are good low carb substitutes for high-carb foods that you used to eat, and you are comfortable with following the Atkins diet for the long haul.

There are no new acceptable foods for phase 4. By this point in time you have added all the foods that you are going to. You should be comfortable with eating foods from each of the 3 phases and you should have found which foods you can and cannot tolerate. And remember, if you start to gain a few pounds back, you can always cut back your net carbs by 10 grams until you lose it and can maintain your weight again.

Of course, as we have said, by this point in time,

Atkins should be a lifestyle. It is not a diet. You should know which foods are good for your long-term maintenance and which is not. By stage 4, you know that life is better on Atkins.

The next chapter outlines a few things to be aware of while following the Atkins diet and how to deal with them.

Chapter 6: Issues to Atkins and How to Avoid Them

As with any diet, there are some things that you should be aware of when following the Atkins diet. Once you are aware of them, you can deal with them effectively.

First, some people do find that they feel weak or lethargic in phase 1 of the Atkins diet. As has already been discussed, you can move to phase 2 fairly quickly, as soon as two weeks after starting the diet. Once you enter phase 2, you will lose weight a little more slowly, but the problems of tiredness and the feeling of deprivation will be less. If you choose to stay in phase 1, make sure that you are getting all of your 20 grams of allotted net carbs. Doing less than this will have adverse effects on how you feel.

Second, being in a state of ketosis can cause bad breath. Make sure to deal with this with mouthwash on a regular basis if you find that you have this problem.

Third, low carb diets may cause constipation in some people. This is because you cut out most of the fiber that your body is used to and fiber is one of the things that help keep your bowels moving. To avoid constipations, there are a couple things you can do. First, make sure to get 12 to 15 grams of net carbs in the foundations vegetables that are listed in phase 1. Those vegetables contain a great deal of fiber and will help keep things moving along well. Second, make sure that you get enough water. If you are dehydrated, you have a much greater chance of developing constipation. Getting at least 64 ounces of water or more will make sure that things keep moving.

One of the drawbacks that a lot of people complain about is that they do not feel that there is enough variety on this diet. Of course, it depends on your point of view. If you are a good cook, there are thousands of recipes out there that you can use on the various phases of this diet that you can make. When you have so many recipes to choose from, the possibilities are endless. Plus, as you move through the phases, your food options increase.

Most people do find phase 1 a struggle, but it becomes less so both when they start to see the weight melt off and as they transition to higher phases, and once they hit lifetime, they are able to eat a wide variety of foods. Included in this book is recipes for each of the four phases, for breakfast, lunch, dinner, and dessert. Once you have tried these foods, you can search the net for more. The options are endless.

The next chapter will list many different recipes for each of the 4 phases.

Chapter 7: Phase 1 recipes

This chapter and the next three will list different recipes for each of the four phases of the Atkins diet. Each phase has 3 breakfast, 3 lunch, 3 dinner, and one dessert recipe. Remember, as you move through the phases, you can eat anything from the previous phase. So if you find a recipe that you like from phase one, you can make it a part of your phase 3 diet.

Breakfast

Flax Meal Muffins

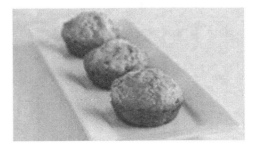

Number of Servings: 1

Ingredients
    1/4 cup flax meal (8.09 total carbs, 7.6 fiber)
    1/2 teaspoon baking powder
    1 packet Splenda packet
    1 teaspoon cinnamon
    1 large egg
    1 teaspoon butter

Directions

- Put the dry ingredients in a coffee mug. Stir.
- Then add the egg and the butter. Mix.
- Microwave 1 minute (or more). Take out. Slice, butter, enjoy. Cream cheese would go nicely, too.

Egg Muffins

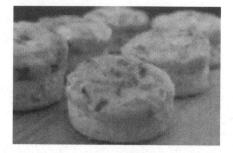

Number of Servings: 12

Ingredients
  15 Large Eggs
  1 Green Bell Pepper
  1 Cup Shredded Cheddar Cheese (low fat if possible)
  1/4 Cup Feta Cheese (Optional)
  Garlic seasoning to taste

Directions

- Preheat oven to 375 F.
- If using a silicone pan, spray with non-stick spray. If using a regular muffin pan, use 2 liners.
- Beat eggs in a bowl. Add diced veggies and cheese. Add garlic seasoning to taste. Pour into muffin tins filling 2/3 full. The muffins will rise.
- Bake 25-35 minutes until muffins have risen and are slightly browned and set.
- Muffins will keep at least a week in the refrigerator without freezing. Egg muffins can be frozen and reheated. For best results, thaw in

refrigerator before reheating. Microwave on high about 2 minutes to reheat.

Cheddar Broccoli Quiche

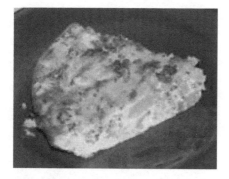

Number of Servings: 6

Ingredients
1 tsp. Canola Oil
1/4 cup finely chopped onion
1 pkg. (10oz) frozen chopped broccoli, thawed, drained.
2 cups egg beaters
1/2 cup low-fat cottage cheese
1/2 cup Kraft 2% shredded reduced fat cheddar cheese
1/8 tsp. black pepper

Directions

- Preheat oven to 350. Heat oil in small nonstick skillet on medium-high heat. Add onions, cook 5 minutes or until onions are tender, stirring occasionally. Add broccoli; mix well. Spoon into 9-in pie plate sprayed with cooking spray.
- Mix remaining ingredients until well blended; pour over broccoli layer.

- Bake 45-50 minutes or until center is set and top is golden brown.

Lunch

Cream of Chicken Soup

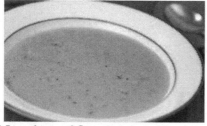

Number of Servings: 1

Ingredients
100g cooked chicken
Celery (allowed amount)
1-2 c broth
3 cloves garlic
1 T dehydrated minced onion
1/2 t parsley
1/2 t basil
Ground white pepper (to taste)
Salt (optional)

Directions

- Preheat saucepan over MED-HI heat.
- In food processor, combine all ingredients and pulse until reaches desired consistency.
- Pour into saucepan and bring to boil.
- Reduce heat to simmer, cover, and heat 20-30 mins.
- Serve

Chili

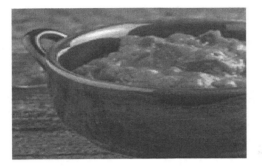

Ingredients

5 lbs. Beef Top Sirloin (Trimmed to 1/8" Fat)
2 tsps. Salt
1/2 tsp Black Pepper
3 tbsps. Extra Virgin Olive Oil
1 medium (2-1/2" dia) Onions
3 tbsps. Chili Powder
14 1/2 oz. Red Tomatoes (with Green Chilies, Canned)
6 fl oz. Red Table Wine
2 tsps. Garlic

Directions

Note: Cooking evaporates alcohol, which is why this recipe is suitable for Induction despite the red wine. But feel free to use chicken broth instead. Jarred roasted garlic cloves can be found in the produce section of most supermarkets.

- Heat oven to 325°F.

Toss beef with salt and pepper. Heat 1 1/2 teaspoons oil in a Dutch oven over high heat. Add one-third of the beef and brown on all sides, about 5 minutes.

- Transfer to a bowl and repeat two more times with beef and oil.
- Chop the onion and add to a Dutch oven preheated with the remaining 1 1/2 teaspoons oil. Cook onion until lightly browned. Stir in chili powder, tomatoes, wine and garlic (minced); bring to a simmer. Return beef and accumulated juices to Dutch oven. Cover and bake 2 1/2 hours, stirring once halfway through cooking time, until beef is very tender. One serving is about 3/4-1 cup.

Buffalo Chicken Egg Salad

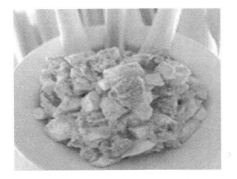

Ingredients

6 large Boiled Eggs
6 oz. boneless, cooked Chicken Thigh
3 tbsps. Real Mayonnaise
1 1/2 tbsps. Red Hot Buffalo Wing Sauce
1/4 cup crumbled Blue or Roquefort Cheese
8 stalk medium (7-1/2" - 8" long) Celery

Directions

Note: Be sure to use a Buffalo hot sauce that has only a few ingredients including red pepper, vinegar and salt; 0g NC per serving.

- Hard boil the eggs: cover 6 eggs with water, bring to a boil, remove from heat and allow to sit for 10 minutes. Immediately plunge eggs into an ice water bath, allow to cool then peel and dice. Reserve in a medium bowl.

- While eggs are cooking cook chicken over medium heat in a skillet or on the grill until the juices run clear and the meat is no longer pink in the center. Cool and dice; add to the eggs in the bowl.

- To the bowl with the diced eggs and chicken add the mayonnaise, Buffalo hot sauce and blue cheese. Mix to combine and blend flavors. Add salt and pepper to taste. Serve with celery stalks for dipping or carefully fill celery stalks. Drizzle with additional Buffalo hot sauce as a garnish or if more heat is desired.

Dinner

Asian Beef Salad Single Serving

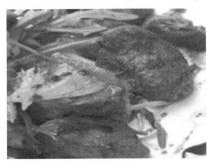

Number of Servings: 1

Ingredients
1/2 clove Garlic
1/2 tbsp. Tamari Soybean Sauce
1/4 tbsp. Sodium and Sugar Free
Rice Vinegar
1/4 tsp Sesame Oil
1/8 tsp Sucralose Based Sweetener (Sugar
Substitute)
1/8 tsp Curry Powder
1/16 tsp Ginger
4 1/4 oz. Beef Top Sirloin (Trimmed to 1/8" Fat,
Choice
Grade)
3/4 cup Spring Mix Salad
1/2 tbsp. Canola Vegetable Oil
1/4 large (2-1/4 per lb., approx. 3-3/4" long,
3" dia) Sweet Red Peppers

Directions

Note: Because only half of the marinade is used in this recipe for the salad dressing and the rest is used as a marinade and discarded, please double the first six ingredients. (The nutritionals shown are correct.). For added flavor, use dark (toasted) sesame oil instead of regular sesame oil.

1. Mix green onions, garlic, soy sauce, rice wine vinegar, sesame oil and sugar substitute in a small bowl. Pour half into a re-sealable plastic bag☐ add steak and marinate overnight in the refrigerator.

2. To remaining soy sauce mixture, add curry powder and ginger. Heat canola oil in a large skillet over high heat until very hot.

3. Drain beef and discard marinade☐ quickly stir-fry beef 2 to 3 minutes in hot oil for medium doneness. Transfer to a large mixing bowl. Add salad greens, bell pepper, water chestnuts and reserved soy dressing. Toss to coat and serve immediately.

Beef Burger with Feta and Tomato

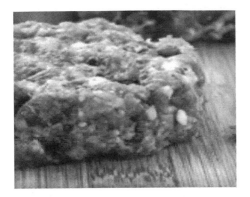

Ingredients
1 lb. Ground Beef (80% Lean / 20% Fat)
1 large Scallions or Spring Onion
1/2 cup Baby Spinach
1/4 cup chopped or sliced Red Tomatoes
1/4 cup crumbled Feta Cheese
1 1/2 tsps. fresh Dill
1/2 tsp Salt
1/2 tsp Black Pepper

Directions
- Combine ground beef, scallion, spinach, tomato, feta, 1.5 tsp fresh dill (or 1/2 tsp dried), salt and pepper. Form into 4 patties.
- Grill or pan-fry over medium-high heat for 6 minutes per side for medium doneness.

Bratwurst with Sauerkraut

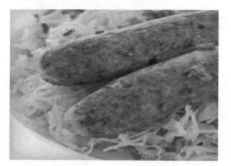

Ingredients
1 stick (3 oz.) Bratwurst
1/2 cup Sauerkraut (Solid and Liquids, Canned)

Directions
- Preheat grill or broiler.
- Grill or broil bratwurst, turning several times until browned on all sides. Or microwave for 1 2 minutes.
- Meanwhile, heat sauerkraut in microwave oven.
- Serve bratwurst with warm sauerkraut.

Dessert

Indulgent Espresso Chocolate Cake

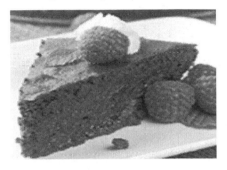

Ingredients
10 oz. Sugar Free Chocolate Chips
10 tbsps. Unsalted Butter Stick
1 tsp rounded Coffee (Instant Powder, Decaffeinated)
1 tbsp. Tap Water
1 tsp Vanilla Extract
1/4 tsp Salt
24 tsps. Erythritol
1 pinch Stevia
4 large Eggs (Whole)
1/3 cup Cocoa Powder (Unsweetened)

Directions
- Preheat oven to 325°F. Grease an 8-inch round baking pan and line with parchment paper (a spring form pan works best). Set aside.

- Melt chocolate and butter in a double boiler. Remove from heat and transfer to a large bowl. Alternatively melt chocolate with butter in a small bowl in the microwave at 30 second intervals; stirring in between. In a small cup, mix espresso powder, water, vanilla and salt; stir into chocolate. Set mixture aside to cool.

- With an electric mixer on medium-high speed, beat eggs, 1/2 cup (24 tsp) granular sugar substitute, stevia and cocoa powder until it falls in thick ribbons when the beater is lifted, about 6 minutes. In three additions, fold eggs into the chocolate mixture.

- Pour batter into prepared pan and smooth top. Bake 30-35 minutes, or until a toothpick inserted near middle of cake comes out with a few moist crumbs and cake is evenly raised. Cool completely on a wire rack. To remove cake, run a knife around edge of pan. Dip bottom of pan into hot water for 1 minute, then turn cake out onto cutting board. (If using a spring form pan, carefully remove sides and serve on the platter.) Turn right side up onto a serving platter.

Chapter 8: Phase 2 recipes

Breakfast

Almond Protein Pancakes

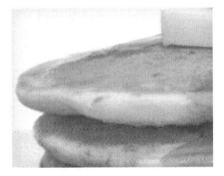

Ingredients
- 2 oz. Vanilla Whey Protein
- 1/4 cup Almond Meal Flour
- 3 tbsps. Whole Grain Soy Flour
- 1 tsp Baking Powder (Straight Phosphate, Double Acting)
- 1/3 cup Large or Small Curd Creamed Cottage Cheese
- 3 large Eggs (Whole)

Directions
Note: Serve with almond butter or sugar-free pancake syrup. Garnish with toasted almonds, if desired.

- Mix the protein powder (1oz is about 4 Tbsp.), almond meal, soy flour and baking powder together. Stir in the beaten eggs and cottage cheese (substitute cream cheese if cottage cheese is not on your accepted foods list) until blended.
- Heat a large non-stick skillet or griddle over medium heat. Lightly grease with butter or canola oil.
- Using about 1/4 cup per pancake, drop batter onto the skillet. When bubbles begin to form in the middle of each pancake, turn over and cook another 2 minutes or until firm.
- Repeat, keeping pancakes warm in the oven.

Almond-Raspberry Smoothie

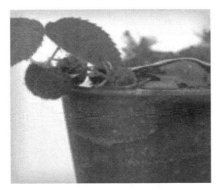

Ingredients

4 oz. Greek Yogurt - Plain (Container)
1/2 cup Red Raspberries
20 whole Blanched & Slivered Almonds
1/2 cup Pure Almond Milk - Unsweetened
Original

Directions

- Feel free to come up with your own combination of other berries and nuts for this protein-packed smoothie. If you use frozen raspberries, make sure they contain no added sugar.
- Combine the yogurt, raspberries, almonds and almond milk in a blender and purée until smooth and creamy.

Baked Eggs and Asparagus

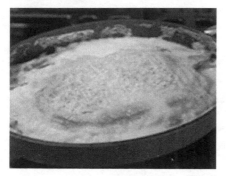

Ingredients

8 spear small (5" long or less) Asparagus
1/4 cup Heavy Cream
2 large Eggs (Whole)
2 tbsps. Almond Meal Flour
1 tbsp. Parmesan Cheese (Shredded)
1/8 tsp Garlic
1/8 tsp Black Pepper

Directions

- Preheat oven to 400°F. Prepare a small oven safe casserole or 4-inch by 3-inch dish with a little bit of oil. Set aside.
- Boil the asparagus spears for 2 minutes until tender-crisp. Drain and run under cold water then pat dry. Arrange in the prepared baking dish.
- Pour cream over the asparagus and then crack two eggs on top.
- In a small bowl blend together the almond meal, Parmesan cheese, garlic and black pepper.

Sprinkle over the eggs and place in the oven. Cook for 5-10 minutes depending upon how you like your eggs cooked. Longer time will result in a firmer yolk. The cream will puff over the edges of the eggs and the topping should be golden brown and fragrant.

Lunch

Asparagus Tarragon Cream Soup

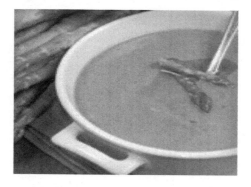

Ingredients

1 tbsp. Extra Virgin Olive Oil
3 14.5 oz. cans Chicken Broth, Bouillon or
Consomme
2 lbs. Asparagus
3 stalk medium (7-1/2" - 8" long) Celery
1/4 tsp Salt
1/4 tsp Black Pepper
1 small Onion
1/2 tbsp. leaf Tarragon
3/4 cup Heavy Cream

Directions

*   Heat oil in a large pot over medium-high heat.
    Add white onion and cook 5 minutes, until
    softened but not browned.

- Add broth, asparagus, celery, salt, pepper and half of the tarragon to the pot. Bring to a boil.
- Lower heat, cover and simmer 20 minutes, until asparagus is very tender.
- In a blender, purée soup in batches until smooth. Return to pot. Add cream and remaining tarragon and heat soup through over medium heat. Season with salt and freshly ground black pepper.

Atkins Cuisine Pizza-Barbecue Chicken Supreme

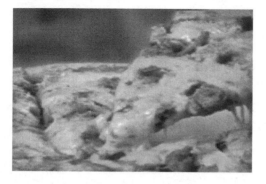

Ingredients

1 1/2 tsps. Baking Powder (Straight Phosphate, Double Acting)
1/2 tsp Salt
1 individual packet Sucralose Based Sweetener (Sugar Substitute)
1 cup Tap Water
1 small Red Onion
1 cup cooked, diced Chicken Breast
2 servings Barbecue Sauce
1/2 medium (approx. 2-3/4" long, 2-1/2" dia) Green Sweet Pepper
6 servings All Purpose Low-Carb Baking Mix
1 cup shredded Whole Milk Mozzarella Cheese
3 tbsps. Extra Virgin Olive Oil

Directions

- Using barbecue sauce instead of tomato sauce spices up the chicken topping. You can substitute other vegetable and meat toppings for variety.
- Heat oven to 425°F.
- Blend together baking mix (2 cups), baking powder, salt and sugar substitute in a large mixing bowl.
- Add water and oil. Using a wooden spoon or a spatula, combine into a dough. Using a spatula, remove the dough from the bowl and place on a clean surface lightly coated with olive oil spray.
- Coat rolling pin with oil spray and roll the dough out to fit the pizza pan or stone. Or use your hands to pat the dough into shape.
- Bake the crust for 10 minutes and remove from oven.
- Spread Barbecue Sauce (about 1/2 cup) evenly over the pizza. Sprinkle with mozzarella and top with chicken pieces, bell pepper slices and onions. Sprinkle with salt and pepper, to taste.
- Return to the oven and continue baking for 10-15 minutes. Cut into 8 slices.

Baked Quesadillas

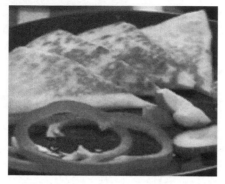

Ingredients

2 tbsps. Light Olive Oil
2 tbsps. chopped Onions
16 oz. Pork Chops or Roasts (Center Rib, Bone-In)
8 slice (1 oz.) Monterey Jack Cheese
1/4 cup Green Tomato Chile Sauce (Salsa Verde)
1 Jalapeno Pepper
1/4 cup Cilantro (Coriander)
1/2 tsp Black Pepper
1/4 tsp Salt
1 tortilla Low Carb Tortillas

Directions

- Make sure the tortillas contain no more than 3 grams of Net Carbs each. Serve with sour cream and additional red or green salsa, if desired.
- Heat oven to 450°F.

- Heat 1 tablespoon of the oil in large skillet over medium-high heat. Cook chopped white onion 5 minutes, until softened.
- Transfer to a bowl. Add pork, cheese, green salsa, chopped jalapeño, cilantro, pepper and salt. Mix well.
- Brush one side of each tortilla with remaining oil.
- Spoon one-sixth of pork mixture over half of non-oiled side of each tortilla and fold in half over filling.
- Place on a baking sheet. Bake 5 minutes, until crisp and golden.

Dinner

Cajun Pork Chops

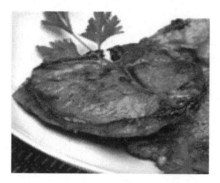

Ingredients

1 tbsp. Paprika
1/2 tsp Cumin
1/2 tsp Sage (Ground)
1/2 tsp Black Pepper
1/2 tsp Garlic Powder
1/2 tsp Red or Cayenne Pepper
24 oz. raw bone-in Pork Chop
1/2 tbsp. Unsalted Butter Stick
1/2 tbsp. Canola Vegetable Oil

Directions

- Combine paprika, cumin, sage, black pepper, garlic powder and cayenne on a plate. Season chops with salt then coat with the seasoning mixture on both sides.

- Heat butter and oil over high heat in a large skillet until very hot. Place chops in skillet, reduce heat to medium and cook 8-9 minutes, turning once halfway through cooking time. Place fish flesh side down in prepared skillet. Bake 10 minutes, turning carefully once halfway through cooking time, until just cooked through.
- Remove from skillet; tent with foil. Add bok choy and lemon peel to skillet. Stir to coat with pan's oil. Place in oven 1 minute, until leaves are wilted and stems are warmed through.
- To make puree, blend peppers and salsa in a blender 30 seconds.
- Top bok choy with fish and dollop with the purée.
- Toss the greens, okra, peppers and snow peas with the Sherry Vinaigrette. Serve with the salmon and bok choy.

Chipotle Grilled Mussels

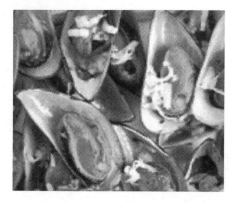

Ingredients

6 tbsps. Unsalted Butter Stick
2 large Scallions or Spring Onions
    2 1/16 peppers with sauces Chipotle Peppers
in Adobo Sauce
1 oz. Cilantro (Coriander)
1 plum Red Tomatoes
2 lbs. Blue Mussels
2 fl oz. Sauvignon Blanc Wine

Directions

• Heat grill to medium. Evenly distribute butter,
  scallions, chipotles, cilantro and tomato on the
  bottom of a large heavy-duty foil cooking bag.
  Add the mussels and wine; tightly seal the bag.
  Place bag on a sheet pan, and refrigerate until grill
  is ready.

• Carefully slide the bag onto grill, and cook until
  the bag is puffed, 10 to 12 minutes. Using oven
  mitts, remove the bag from grill, placing it back

onto sheet pan. Carefully unseal the bag (steam will be released) to check that the mussels have opened. If not, reseal, and cook 3 to 5 minutes more.

- Remove from grill, and carefully cut the bag open, pulling back the foil. Serve immediately, spooning juice in bag over mussels.

Cornish Hens with Apricot Glaze

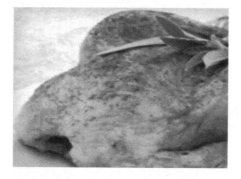

Ingredients

4 bird wholes Chicken Meat (Cornish Game Hens)
1/2 tsp Salt
1/4 tsp Black Pepper
1/2 tsp Cinnamon
1/4 tsp ground Cardamom
1 tbsp. Extra Virgin Olive Oil
2 tbsps. chopped Shallots
1 cup Chicken Broth, Bouillon or Consomme
8 tbsps. Sugar Free Apricot Preserves
2 tsps. Thick-It-Up

Directions

- Heat oven to 450°F.
- Rinse hens under cold running water and then drain and blot dry with paper towels. Place one hen on its breast. With poultry shears make a lengthwise cut down one side of the backbone to

the tail. Repeat on other side of backbone; remove and discard backbone. Remove and discard fat inside the body and neck cavities. Place hen cut-side down and flatten with your hands. Transfer to a baking sheet. Repeat with remaining hens. Sprinkle with salt and pepper.

- In a small bowl, mix jam, cinnamon and cardamom.
- Cook 25 minutes, until no longer pink inside and juices run clear. Heat broiler. Brush reserved glaze on hens. Broil 6 from heat source 2 minutes, until browned. Remove from broiler. Transfer hens to a serving platter; tent with foil to keep warm.
- In skillet over medium heat, heat olive oil. Add shallots and cook 2 minutes, stirring occasionally, until softened. Carefully pour accumulated juices from the baking sheet into skillet. Add chicken broth. Bring to a boil over medium-high heat. Whisk in thickener. Simmer 1 minute until thickened. Transfer sauce to a gravy boat and serve immediately.

Dessert

Extra-Creamy Strawberry Shake

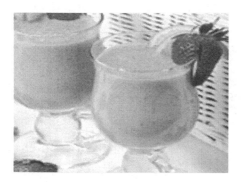

Ingredients

  6 medium (1-1/4" dia) Strawberries
  2 scoops Strawberry Whey Protein
  1/2 cup Heavy Cream
  1 tsp Vanilla Extract
  2 cups Tap Water
    2 individual packets Sucralose Based
  Sweetener (Sugar Substitute)

Directions

* Place strawberries, protein mix, cream, vanilla,
  water, and sugar substitute in a blender and blend
  at high speed until very smooth.

Chapter 9: Phase 3 recipes

Breakfast

California Breakfast Burrito

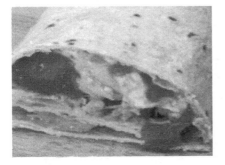

Ingredients

4 tortillas Low Carb Tortillas
1 tbsp. Canola Vegetable Oil
3 large Scallions or Spring Onions
4 oz. Green Chili Peppers (Canned)
1 medium whole (2-3/5" dia) Red Tomatoes
1/2 tsp Salt
1/4 tsp Black Pepper
8 large Eggs (Whole)
1/8 tsp Red or Cayenne Pepper
9 sprigs Cilantro (Coriander)
1/2 cup shredded Cheddar Cheese
1 serving Tomatillo Salsa

Directions

- Use 1/4 cup total of the Atkins recipe for Tomatillo Salsa.
- Heat oven to 325° F.
- Wrap tortillas in foil and heat in oven 5-10 minutes. Chop tomatoes and dice green onions.
- In a medium non-stick skillet, heat oil over medium-high heat. Add green onions, chilies, tomato, salt and pepper. Sauté for 3 minutes.
- Push mixture to side of pan. Add eggs and cayenne to skillet. Cook, 1-2 minutes, stirring occasionally with rubber spatula, until soft, creamy curds form.
- Stir vegetable mixture into eggs.
- Divide mixture among warm tortillas, sprinkle with cilantro, one tablespoon of salsa and 2 tablespoons cheese. Roll up tortillas.

Cinnamon Buns

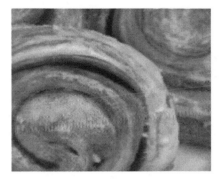

Ingredients

1 1/2 tsps. Baking Powder (Straight Phosphate,
Double Acting)
1/2 tsp Salt
1/2 cup Unsalted Butter Stick
2 large Egg Yolks
1 1/2 cups Tap Water
1 tsp Cinnamon
6 tbsps. Sucralose Based Sweetener (Sugar
Substitute)
1/2 cup chopped Pecans
1 1/2 oz. Dried Currants
1 tbsp. Heavy Cream
6 servings All Purpose Low-Carb Baking Mix
5 1/4 tbsps. Sugar Free Brown Sugar Cinnamon
Syrup

Low-Carb Baking Mix:
All Purpose Low-Carb Baking Mix

Ingredients
1/4 cup Wheat Bran (Crude)
1 1/8 cups Whole Grain Soy Flour
2/3 cup Vanilla Whey Protein
1/4 cup Organic 100% Whole Ground Golden
Flaxseed Meal
2/3 cup Vital Wheat Gluten Flour

Directions
Note: It is not necessary to use vanilla flavored whey
protein powder, unflavored is ideal but the vanilla
will not contribute much flavor to the mix so if it is
what you have on hand, use it.

• Combine all ingredients and mix thoroughly. Use
  immediately or store in an airtight container in the
  refrigerator for up to 1 month. Each recipe
  makes 9 servings or 3 cups. Each serving size is
  1/3 cup.

Directions

• In a large bowl mix baking mix (you will need 2
  cups of the above recipe), baking powder, salt,
  water, 4 tablespoons butter, 4 tablespoons sugar
  substitute and 1 egg yolk until smooth. Cover
  lightly with plastic wrap and let rise one hour.
  Stretch dough out to a rectangle measuring 10x15
  inches, long side facing towards you.

- For filling: mix 4 tablespoons butter, 2 tablespoons sugar substitute and cinnamon. Brush mixture over dough, leaving a ½ border at the bottom. Sprinkle dough evenly with nuts and currants. Roll dough up lengthwise from the top, stretching it as you go along. Pinch dough tightly to seal roll and pat to even out shape if necessary. Cut dough roll in half, then halve each half, then cut each quarter into thirds (you will have 12 even slices). Arrange slices on a nonstick baking sheet, lightly cover with plastic wrap and let rise 45 minutes. Heat oven to 375°F.

- Mix 1 egg yolk and cream. Brush dough slices with mixture. Bake 30 to 35 minutes until lightly browned. Cool buns five minutes then brush with sugar-free cinnamon syrup. Serve warm or at room temperature.

French Quesadillas

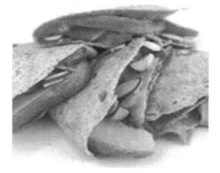

Ingredients

3 oz. boneless, cooked Fresh Ham
1 medium (approx. 2-1/2 per lb.) Pears
4 tortillas Low Carb Tortillas
4 oz. Brie Cheese
1/4 cup sliced Almonds

Directions

- Preheat oven to 350°F.
- Lay tortillas flat onto a sheet pan. Layer onto half of each tortilla the pear, ham, Brie cheese and almonds (in that order).
- Fold the tortilla over and bake for 5 minutes; cut in half and enjoy immediately.

Lunch

Fresh Mozzarella, Haricots Vert and Tomato Salad

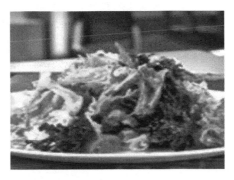

Ingredients

1/2 lb. Green Snap Beans
4 pieces Marinated Artichoke Hearts
2 plums Red Tomatoes
6 oz. Fresh Mozzarella
1/4 cup chopped English Walnuts
2/3 tbsp. Red Wine Vinegar
1/2 tsp Dijon Mustard
1/2 tsp Salt
1/4 tsp Black Pepper
3 tbsps. Extra Virgin Olive Oil

Directions

- Bring a large pot of lightly salted water to a boil. Add beans and cook until crisp-tender, 6 to 8 minutes. Drain and rinse under cold water.

- Place two artichoke hearts in the center of each of two plates. Circle each with half of the tomato slices. Arrange half of the green beans and half of the cheese slices around the artichokes on each plate. Sprinkle with the walnuts, if desired.
- Make the dressing: in a small bowl, whisk together the vinegar, mustard, salt, pepper and oil until well combined. Spoon dressing over salad and serve.

Italian Sausage Morning Soup

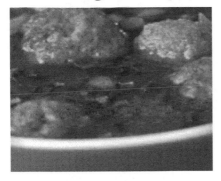

Ingredients

1 tbsp. Extra Virgin Olive Oil
1/2 cup chopped Onions
1 stalk medium (7-1/2" - 8" long) Celery
1/2 cup chopped Carrots
4 cups Chicken Broth, Bouillon or Consomme
1/4 cup Spaghetti/Marinara Pasta Sauce
1/4 tsp Italian Seasoning
8 oz. cooked Italian Sausage
4 oz. Ground Beef (80% Lean / 20% Fat)
1 large Egg (Whole)

Directions

- Heat olive oil in a large saucepan over medium heat. Add the white onion, celery and carrots and cook until they begin to soften, about 5 minutes.
- Add the broth, marinara sauce and Italian seasoning. Simmer for 20 minutes.

- Meanwhile, mix the sausage, ground beef and egg together in a mixing bowl. Using a tablespoon, form meat mixture into balls and drop into the simmering soup. Alternatively, bake the meatballs in a 350°F oven on a jelly roll pan until brown on the outside before adding to the soup.
- Cook for an additional 20 minutes until the meatballs are cooked through.
- Season to taste with salt and freshly ground pepper and serve immediately.

Mexican Shrimp and Vegetable Salad

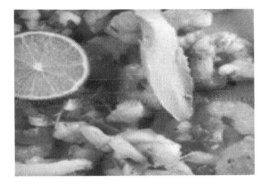

Ingredients

4 medium Turnips
1 medium Carrot
3 tbsps. Extra Virgin Olive Oil
3/4 cup Green Tomato Chile Sauce (Salsa Verde)
2 lbs. Shrimp
1 medium whole (2-3/5" dia) Red Tomatoes
1 head (5" dia) Butterhead Lettuce (Includes Boston and Bibb Types)
1 fruit without skin and seed California Avocado
1/4 cup Cilantro (Coriander)

Directions

- In a medium saucepan, cook turnips and carrot in lightly salted boiling water 7 to 8 minutes, until crisp-tender. Drain and rinse under cold water. Pat dry.
- Heat oil in a large skillet over medium-high heat. Add salsa and cook 5 minutes, until slightly thickened. Add shrimp and cook 2 minutes. Stir

in tomato and vegetables; cook 2 minutes more until shrimp are just cooked and vegetables are heated through.

- Arrange lettuce leaves on individual serving plates. Top with shrimp mixture; garnish with sliced avocado and cilantro.

Dinner

Creamy Coconut Curried Chicken

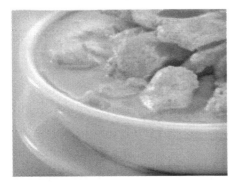

Ingredients

4 tbsps. Canola Vegetable Oil
2 tbsps. Curry Powder
1 tsp Cumin
3 tsps. Ginger
2 tbsps. Tomato Paste
2 1/4 cups Chicken Broth, Bouillon or Consomme
64 oz. boneless, cooked Chicken Breast
1 cup Coconut Cream
1 small Onion
1/2 tbsp. Sour Cream (Cultured)
1 1/4 tbsps. Baby Spinach
1 oz. Cilantro (Coriander)
1/2 serving All Purpose Low-Carb Baking Mix
9 tsps. Garlic

Directions

Use the recipe to make Low-Carb Baking Mix for this recipe. (See breakfast recipe Cinnamon Buns in Phase 3)

- Heat oil in large saucepot or Dutch oven over medium heat. Sauté onion until golden, about 5 minutes. Add garlic, curry, cumin and ginger and sauté for another minute. Add tomato paste and sauté for another minute. Add baking mix and cook, stirring constantly, about 1 minute. Slowly whisk in broth, increase heat to high and bring to a boil. Reduce heat to low and simmer 20 minutes, stirring occasionally, until sauce thickens slightly.
- Add chicken to pot, and simmer 10 to 2 minutes, until chicken is just cooked through. Whisk in coconut milk and sour cream and return to a simmer just to heat through (do not boil). Turn off heat and stir in spinach until it starts to wilt. Season with salt and pepper and sprinkle with cilantro before serving. Top with coconut and peanuts, if desired.

Fried Hazelnut-Crusted Calamari with Spicy Tomato Sauce

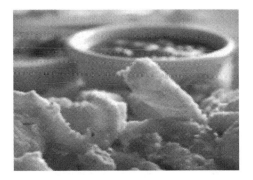

Ingredients

1 tbsp. Extra Virgin Olive Oil
1 tbsp. Parsley
1 1/3 cups Tomato Sauce (Canned)
1 cup chopped Hazelnuts or Filberts
1/4 tsp Crushed Red Pepper Flakes
1 lb. Squid (Mixed Species)
1/4 tsp Chili Powder
1/4 cup Peanut Oil
1/8 tsp Salt
2 servings All Purpose Low-Carb Baking Mix
1 fruit (2-1/8" dia) Lemon

Directions

- Use the s recipe to make Low-Carb Baking Mix for this recipe. (See breakfast recipe Cinnamon Buns in Phase 3)
- Use 2 cups oil for frying in this recipe.

- For sauce: In a large skillet, heat olive oil over medium heat. Add parsley and red pepper flakes and sauté for 1 minute. Add tomato sauce and bring to a simmer. Cook, stirring occasionally, for 5 minutes (sauce may be made up to two days in advance).
- In a food processor, process hazelnuts, 2/3 cups baking mix and cayenne until nuts are finely ground, about 1 minute. Transfer to a shallow bowl. Dredge calamari in mixture, tapping to remove any excess, and set aside.
- Heat oil in a deep sauce pot until temperature reaches 375°F. Fry calamari in batches, 30 seconds per batch, until firm and light golden. Transfer to a paper-towel-lined plate to drain. Sprinkle with salt and serve with sauce and lemon wedges.

Low-carb Lasagna

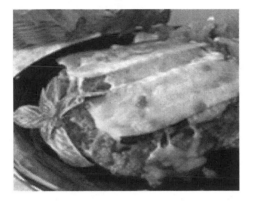

Ingredients
2 medium Zucchinis
1/2 lb. Ground Beef (80% Lean / 20% Fat)
1/4 cup chopped Onions
1 1/4 cup chopped or sliced Red Tomatoes
1 can (6 oz.) Tomato Paste
1/2 tsp Garlic
1/2 tsp leaf Oregano
1 large Egg (Whole)
1/2 tsp leaf Basil (Dried)
1/4 tsp leaf Dried Thyme Leaves
1/4 cup Tap Water
1/8 tsp Black Pepper
3/4 cup Large or Small Curd Creamed Cottage Cheese
1/2 cup shredded Mozzarella Cheese (Whole Milk)
1/16 cup 100% Stone Ground Whole Wheat Pastry Flour

Directions

- Cook zucchini until tender, drain and set aside.
- Fry meat and onions until meat is brown and onions are tender; drain fat. Add next 8 ingredients and bring to a boil. Reduce heat; simmer, uncovered 10 minutes or until reduced to 2 cups.
- In a small bowl slightly beat egg. Add cottage cheese, half of shredded cheese and flour.
- In a 1 1/2-qt. baking/roasting pan arrange half of the meat mixture. Top with half of the zucchini and all the cottage cheese mixture. Top with remaining meat and zucchini. Bake uncovered at 375°F for 30 minutes. Sprinkle with remaining cheese and bake 10 minutes longer. Let stand for 10 minutes before serving.

Dessert

Fresh Berry Tarts with Cream

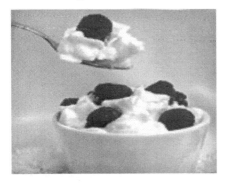

Ingredients

2/3 cup, slivered Almonds
1/2 cup Fresh Blueberries
1/4 cup Heavy Cream
1/2 cup Red Raspberries
2 tbsps. Sucralose Based Sweetener (Sugar Substitute)

Directions

- Heat broiler. Chop almonds and divide among 4 small ramekins. Sprinkle 1 tablespoon sugar substitute over the almonds. Place ramekins on a cookie sheet and broil until the tops of the nuts are golden and the sugar substitute has melted. Remove and cool until at room temperature.

- Whip the heavy cream and remaining tablespoon of sugar substitute until doubled in volume. Place one-quarter of blueberries and one-quarter of raspberries in each ramekin and top with a dollop of whipped cream. Serve immediately.

Chapter 10: Phase 4 recipes

Breakfast

Farmers Breakfast Soup

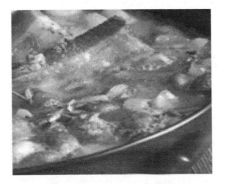

Ingredients

1/2 cup chopped Onions
2 medium slice (yield after cooking) Bacon
8 oz. Turkey Sausage
4 oz. Ground Beef (80% Lean / 20% Fat)
2/3 cup High Protein TVP (Textured Vegetable Protein)
1/2 cup chopped Celery
1/2 cup chopped Carrots
4 cups Chicken Broth, Bouillon or Consomme
1/4 tsp Black Pepper

Directions

- In a large non-stick skillet, over medium heat, cook the bacon until it begins to brown. Add the sausage and beef to brown, breaking up the meat into small bits with a spatula or spoon (about 7 minutes).
- Stir in the TVP and vegetables. Cook 5 minutes until vegetables begin to soften.
- Add remaining ingredients and simmer for 20 minutes, skimming off excess fat from the surface of the liquid.
- Season with salt and pepper to taste.

Mini Chocolate Chip Muffins

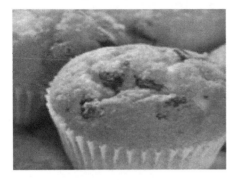

Ingredients

1 cup Whole Grain Soy Flour
1 tsp Baking Powder (Straight Phosphate, Double Acting)
1/2 cup Sucralose Based Sweetener (Sugar Substitute)
1/4 tsp Salt
1/2 cup Sour Cream (Cultured)
2 tbsps. Unsalted Butter Stick
2 tbsps. Heavy Cream
1 fl oz. Tap Water
2 tsps. Vanilla Extract
4 oz. Sugar Free Chocolate Chips

Directions

- Heat oven to 350°F. Grease two 12-compartment mini muffin pans.
- In a bowl, combine soy flour, baking powder, sugar substitute, and salt.

- In another bowl, whisk sour cream, butter, heavy cream, water and vanilla to combine.
- Add the sour cream mixture to the soy mixture. Stir until well combined. Fold in chocolate chips.
- Divide batter (it will be somewhat thick) in pan compartments, using about 1 rounded tablespoon per muffin. Bake 15-20 minutes, or until lightly browned on top and toothpick inserted in center comes out clean.
- Cool muffins in pans for 2 minutes, then turn out onto wire racks to cool completely.

Power "Oatmeal"

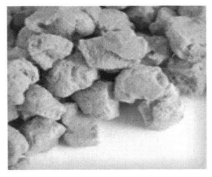

Ingredients

3 oz. Dry Textured Vegetable Protein
1 14 oz. can Coconut Cream
1 cup Tap Water
1/4 tsp Cinnamon
     1/2 cup Large or Small Curd Creamed
Cottage Cheese
2 oz. Vanilla Whey Protein

Directions

Note: You can find textured vegetable protein (TVP)
in any natural foods store or in some well-stocked
supermarkets. In this recipe its texture suggests
oatmeal.

- Combine the textured vegetable protein, coconut
  milk, water, cinnamon, protein powder and
  cottage cheese in a large saucepan with a heavy
  bottom.

- Cook, over low heat, for 20 minutes, or until mixture has thickened and is tender. Serve with a little cream and sugar substitute, if desired.

Lunch

Blueberry-Turkey Burgers

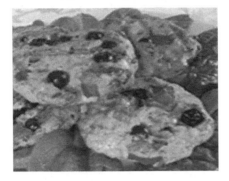

Ingredients

1 1/4 lbs. Ground Turkey
1 tbsp. Light Olive Oil
3 tbsps. Peppermint (Mint)
1 1/2 tsps. Fennel Seed
1 1/2 tsps. Cumin
1/2 tsp Salt
1/2 tsp Black Pepper
1/2 cup chopped Red Sweet Pepper
3/4 cup crumbled Feta Cheese
3/4 cup Blueberries

Directions

- Ground turkey can be dry, adding additional olive oil is optional but the bell pepper and blueberries may pop out more easily. Use ground lamb for a different flavor.

- Using your hands combine the ground turkey, olive oil, chopped mint, ground fennel, ground cumin, salt and pepper in a medium bowl.
- Add the chopped red bell peppers, feta cheese and blueberries gently combining and then form into 6 equal burgers. The blueberries or peppers may need to be popped back into the burgers. Simply push them gently into place on the top side. Season with additional salt and freshly ground black pepper.
- Grill or pan fry over medium-high heat until the internal temperature reaches 165°F and the meat is no longer pink in the center and the juices run clear. Serve immediately.

Bones-to-Be Chicken Wingettes

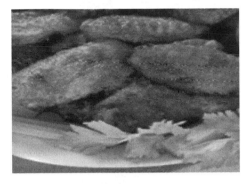

Ingredients

2 tbsps. Chili Powder
1 tsp Red or Cayenne Pepper
2 tsps. Yellow Mustard Seed
2 tsps. Salt
1/2 serving All Purpose Low-Carb Baking Mix
32 oz., with bone (yield after cooking, bone removed) Chicken Wing

Directions

Note: Use the Atkins recipe to make All Purpose Low-Carb Baking Mix for this recipe. You will need half of a 1/3 cup (about 3 Tbsp.) = half of a serving.

- Heat oven to 450°F. Line a jelly-roll pan with foil, and spray with nonstick cooking spray.
- Combine chili powder, 2 Tbsp. baking mix, cayenne, mustard and salt in a large resealable bag. Add half of the wingettes, and shake to coat. Transfer to pan, and repeat with remaining wingettes.

- Bake, turning occasionally, until crisp, browned and cooked through, 30 to 35 minutes. Transfer to a platter, and serve.

Chicken Soup with Dilled Mini-Matzo Balls

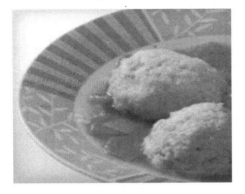

Ingredients

24 oz. boneless, cooked Chicken Thigh
3 14.5 oz. cans Chicken Broth, Bouillon or Consomme
4 1/2 cups Tap Water
1 small Red Onion
5 small (5-1/2" long) Carrots
1 stalk medium (7-1/2" - 8" long) Celery
1 1/2 tsps. Garlic
6 sprigs Parsley
1/2 oz. Dill
1/4 tsp leaf Dried Thyme Leaves
1/2 tsp Black Pepper
1 large Egg (Whole)
1 tbsp. Canola Vegetable Oil
1 medium (4-1/8" long) Scallions or Spring Onions
1/4 cup Matzo Meal

Directions

- For the soup: Combine chicken, broth, water, onion, carrot, celery and garlic in a large saucepan. Bring to a boil over high heat. Skim off foam that rises to surface. Add parsley, dill, thyme and peppercorns; reduce heat to very low and simmer gently until flavors develop, about 1 1/2 hours.
- Transfer chicken to a cutting board. Strain broth into a clean container; skim off fat and season with salt and pepper to taste. Discard solids. Remove and discard skin from chicken; pull meat off bones and return to broth.
- For the matzo balls: Combine egg, oil, dill and scallion in a small bowl. Beat with a fork, then stir in matzo ball mix until well blended. Cover and refrigerate for 15 minutes.
- Meanwhile, bring a large pot of salted water to a boil over high heat. With wet hands, shape matzo mixture into 16 balls using 1 level teaspoon for each, and drop balls into water. Reduce heat to low; cover and simmer until cooked through, about 15 minutes. Reheat soup. With a slotted spoon, transfer matzo balls to soup and serve.

Dinner

Fresh Salmon Cakes with Avocado Tartar Sauce

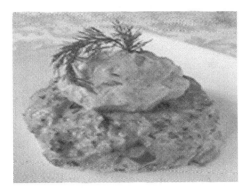

Ingredients

1 fruit without skin and seed California Avocado
16 oz. boneless Salmon
    1/2 medium (approx. 2-3/4" long, 2-1/2"
dia) Red Sweet Pepper
2 stalk medium (7-1/2" - 8" long) Celery
1 tsp Original Stone Ground Mustard
5 tbsps. Real Mayonnaise
1 tbsp. drained Capers
1/4 cup Parsley
1 large Egg (Whole)
2 tsps. Old Bay Seasoning
1 tbsp. Fresh Lemon Juice
2 tsps. fresh Dill

Directions

- Preheat oven to 450°F. Prepare a baking sheet with a small amount of oil in 4 spots about 6 inches apart. Set aside.
- Coarsely chop the red pepper and celery. Skin salmon if skin is intact and chop into 4-inch pieces. Place all into a food processor. A food processor is not required, just be sure to finely chop all ingredients before combining (including the capers and parsley below).
- Add the mustard, 2 tablespoons mayonnaise, capers, parsley, egg and Old Bay seasoning. Pulse 4-5 times just until the salmon is chopped. Season with salt and freshly ground black pepper. Using a 2/3 cup measuring scoop - divide the mixture into 4 equal rounded mounds on the prepared baking sheet.
- Cook for 20 minutes and move to serving plates. Garnish each cake with 2 Tablespoons avocado tartar sauce.
- Avocado Tartar Sauce: combine the avocado, 3 tablespoons mayonnaise, lemon juice and chopped dill in a blender (or mash by hand). Blend until smooth adding salt and black pepper to taste. 2 heaping tablespoons per serving.

Mini Italian Meatloaves

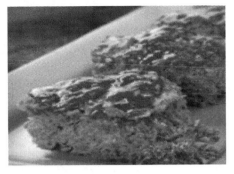

Ingredients

    1 1/2 lbs. Ground Beef (80% Lean / 20% Fat)
    12 oz. raw (yield after cooking) Italian Sausage
    5 pieces Dried Porcini Mushrooms
    1/4 cup Dried Pine Nuts
    2 large Eggs (Whole)
    1/2 tsp Italian Seasoning
    2 cups Spinach
    2 1/2 oz. Spaghetti/Marinara Pasta Sauce

Directions

- Preheat oven to 350°F.
- Mist 4 mini-loaf pans with olive-oil spray. Set aside.
- Rehydrate mushrooms in 1/2 cup hot water, allow to sit for 10 minutes, then drain.
- In a large mixing bowl, thoroughly combine ground beef seasoned with salt and freshly ground black pepper, chopped sausage, re-hydrated

mushrooms, beaten eggs, pine nuts, herbs and chopped spinach.

- Divide into four equal portions and press into greased loaf pans. Drizzle 1 tablespoon marinara sauce on top of each and place on a baking sheet. Bake for 50 minutes.

- Remove from oven and let rest for 10 minutes before serving.

Red Snapper, Vegetable and Pesto Packets

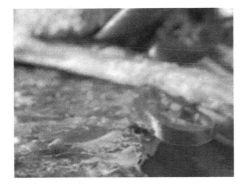

Ingredients

4 medium (4 1/8" long) Scallions or Spring
Onions
1/2 cup Pesto Sauce
1 tbsp. Extra Virgin Olive Oil
1/2 tsp Salt
1 1/2 lbs. Snapper (Fish) (Mixed Species)
12 spear medium (5-1/4" to 7" long) Asparagus
2 small Yellow Summer Squashes
1 tbsp. Fresh Lemon Juice
1 small (5 per pound) Red Sweet Pepper
2 tbsps. Pine Nuts

Directions

- Heat oven to 425°F.
- Combine Basil Pesto, lemon juice, olive oil and
  salt in a large bowl. Gently spread half the mixture
  on fish, and toss vegetables with remaining
  mixture to coat.

- Cut four 12 x 12 squares heavy-duty aluminum foil; fold each square in half, then open again. Distribute vegetables evenly over one side of each square, leaving a 1 border; lay one fillet on top of each. Sprinkle with pine nuts.
- Seal and crimp edges to make packets. Transfer packets to a baking sheet, and bake 25 minutes. Open packets directly on dinner plates.

Dessert

Holiday Gingerbread

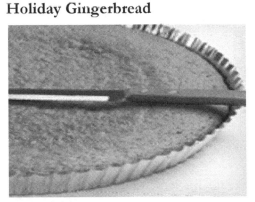

Ingredients

1/2 tsp Cinnamon
1 tsp Baking Powder (Straight Phosphate, Double Acting)
1/2 tsp Salt
1/4 tsp Cloves (Ground)
1 tsp Nutmeg (Ground)
1/2 cup 100% Stone Ground Whole Wheat Pastry Flour
9 tbsps. Sucralose Based Sweetener (Sugar Substitute)
8 large Eggs (Whole)
3 tsps. Ginger
1/4 cup Unsalted Butter Stick
1/2 cup Heavy Cream
1/2 tsp Ginger (Ground)
1 fl oz. Coffee (Brewed From Grounds)

1 1/2 servings All Purpose Low-Carb Baking Mix
3 tbsps. Cocoa Powder (Unsweetened)

Directions

Note: Use the Atkins recipe to make All Purpose
Low-Carb Baking Mix for this recipe.

- Heat oven to 350°F. Butter a 9-inch round cake pan.
- Whisk flour, 1/2 cup baking mix, cocoa powder, baking powder, salt, nutmeg, cinnamon, ground ginger and cloves in a bowl to combine.
- In another bowl, beat egg yolks and sugar substitute with an electric mixer on high speed until thick ribbons form when the beaters are lifted, 3 to 4 minutes. Beat in butter until smooth. Add cream, fresh ginger and coffee; beat until thoroughly combined, about 1 minute.
- With a clean mixing bowl and beaters, beat egg whites until stiff peaks form, 3 to 4 minutes. Mix one-third of egg whites into batter to lighten. Gently fold in remaining egg whites in two additions until just combined. Pour batter into prepared pan.
- Bake until cake has risen and a toothpick inserted in the center comes out clean, 22- to 25 minutes. Cool cake in pan on a wire rack for 5 minutes. Remove cake from pan and let cool completely on the rack.
- If desired, whip extra cream flavored with ground ginger and sugar substitute to taste. Serve gingerbread with a dollop of flavored whipped cream.

Chapter 11: Example Meal Plan

This chapter will give you a sample meal plan for several days of the induction phase 1 of the Atkins diet. Once you have a handle on the induction phase, it will be easier for you to add foods to your diet. Because it is usually phase 1 that most people struggle with, this is the one that we are including as a sample meal plan.

Day 1:

Breakfast: 2 eggs and a slice of cheese

Lunch: cheeseburger (no bun), lettuce, mayo, pickle

Dinner: grilled chicken legs, salad

Snack: Hard-boiled egg, 1 small tomato

Day 2:

Breakfast: Eggs and mushrooms (see recipe)

Lunch: Leftover chicken legs, salad, green pepper, onion

Dinner: recipe from phase 1 (whichever you like)

Snack: 1 Stick Mozzarella string cheese

Day 3:

Breakfast: Egg muffin (see recipe)

Lunch: Chili (see recipe), ½ cup yellow squash

Dinner: Chipless beef nachos

Snack: A variety of vegetables from the foundation list

Day 4:

Breakfast: Flax muffins (see recipe), side veggies, hard-boiled egg

Lunch: Cream of mushroom soup, piece of chicken, salad

Dinner: Pork chop, cauliflower, salad with dressing

Snack: Serving of Swiss cheese and cucumber

As you can see, adding foods to the meal plan is easy. The key is to make sure that you get 4 to 6 ounces of a protein in each meal (eggs and meats), make sure that you have vegetables, and get your 20 grams total net carbs. You can add or subtract foods as you like.

Conclusion:

Congratulations! By reading these books, you have taken the first step to having a better life through a healthy diet and weight loss program. Instead of dieting, you have learned to make changes that can last a lifetime. And the Atkins diet is a healthy alternative to eating processed foods and carbs that are keeping the fat on and making you unhappy. By following this plan, you will lose weight quickly. In fact, you can lose up to 30 pounds in

30 days by following Atkins! You now have all the tools that you need to make an effective change in your life. So what are you waiting for? Now is the time to take control of your eating and control of your life!

You may also like these books...

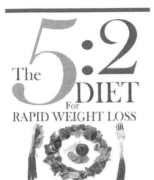

The 5:2 DIET For RAPID WEIGHT LOSS

Lose Weight Fast Using Intermittent Fasting And Look Great Without Trying

FlatBelly Queens

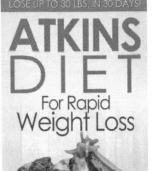

LOSE UP TO 30 LBS. IN 30 DAYS!

ATKINS DIET For Rapid Weight Loss

FlatBelly Queens

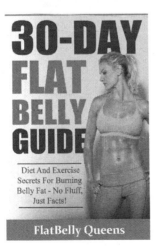

30-DAY FLAT BELLY GUIDE

Diet And Exercise Secrets For Burning Belly Fat - No Fluff, Just Facts!

FlatBelly Queens

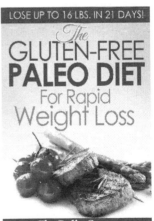

LOSE UP TO 16 LBS. IN 21 DAYS!

The GLUTEN-FREE PALEO DIET For Rapid Weight Loss

FlatBelly Queens

Made in the USA
San Bernardino, CA
05 February 2018